COMMUNITY PARTICIPATION IN HEALTH PROMOTION

COMMUNITY PARTICIPATION IN HEALTH PROMOTION

Jan Smithies and Lee Adams, Health Education Authority
with Georgina Webster and Alan Beattie

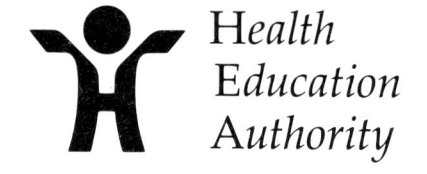

Health
Education
Authority

Published in 1990
Health Education Authority
Hamilton House
Mabledon Place
London WC1H 9TX

ISBN 1 85448 084 7

These materials were originally produced for the fourth annual Healthy Cities Symposium held in Pécs, Hungary, in September 1989

Printed and bound in Great Britain by
Biddles Ltd, Guildford and King's Lynn

Contents

Preface		6
Introduction		7
Section 1:	Keywords and Definitions	9
Section 2:	Case Studies	16
Section 3:	Structured Bibliography	46
Section 4:	Summary	61
Section 5:	Key Texts: a useful starting point	62

Preface

We initially devised, wrote and edited this publication, at the invitation of the Health Promotion Unit, WHO Copenhagen, to support the 1989 Healthy Cities Symposium held in Pécs (Hungary), and to promote on-going community action work within Healthy Cities. However demand for copies of the publication in the UK has now exceeded our capacity to photocopy it, so it is now appropriate to publish it for a UK audience.

We would like to acknowledge the substantial contributions of Alan Beattie of Lancaster University, who compiled the Bibliography, and Georgina Webster, Freelance Trainer and Consultant, who compiled the Case Studies section.

We would also like to thank the Health Education Authority staff who have worked with us on the production of the booklet and all the individuals and projects who contributed time, support and information.

Lee Adams
Jan Smithies
Professional and Community Development Division of the Health Education Authority, Hamilton House, Mabledon Place, London WC1H 9TX, England.

January 1990

Introduction

Community participation in health has developed its own discrete identity in the UK over the last 10 years with the emergence of 'community health projects'; a new professional group – 'community health workers' and the setting up of a national voluntary organisation – the 'National Community Health Resource', responsible for supporting and promoting local and national community action and development on health issues.

The last two years have also seen the emergence of statutory National Health Service support for community development in health education through the setting up of our own division for 'Professional and Community Development' within the Health Education Authority, and some similar initiatives in local and regional Health and Local Authorities throughout the country.

Here in the UK, community participation has roots that go back well into history. The basis of many of the major changes in health and public policy, service provision and legislation can be traced back to some form of community pressure and/or participation.

The 1980s have seen the formal linking of community development and health issues, resulting in a significant social movement for change which has developed through local, regional and national projects and forums and operates through both formal and informal channels and networks. This social movement includes unpaid activists, volunteers, community workers, community health workers, primary health care workers, some planners and policy makers, academics and researchers, health promotion workers and community physicians. However the main impetus still remains at present with voluntary and community groups. The movement has three basic 'Health for All' principles – increasing community participation, encouraging more collaboration between statutory and voluntary sectors, and highlighting and reducing inequalities in health.

Healthy Cities initiatives, pioneered by the WHO European Office in Copenhagen, are a clear example of health promotion activity both in terms of strategy and practice. They are now themselves developing into local, regional, national and international social movements and need to continue to forge strong connections and links with the community participation and community health movements in all their many forms.

The skills, experience and concepts that have been built up by paid workers and voluntary activists can contribute a great deal to Healthy Cities, and other major health promotion activities, and help accelerate the progress of community awareness and participation at all levels in planning, policy development and action for health.

We hope the projects and references included here will help clarify connections, stimulate new ideas and work, and create practical openings for international debate on the importance of putting into practice community participation in 'Health For All' work.

This publication is mainly based on the UK experience and we realise that in many other countries concepts such as self-help and community action do not necessarily have the same meanings and definitions. Nor is the divide between Local Authority, Health Authority and Voluntary Sector conceptually and organisationally the same as in the UK. We have tried wherever possible to explain the context of projects in Section 2 to make it accessible to an international audience. Likewise Section 1 provides key words and definitions to help readers clarify the terminology used in the later sections of the publication, and to assist with international comparisons of concepts.

The Bibliography (Section 3) is again heavily UK-based, but we hope colleagues from other countries will add their own references and texts to develop this into an international resource on community participation in health.

There are of course dangers in institutionalising community participation and it is important that there are those of us working from the 'inside' to open up possibilities for participation, and people on the 'outside' who are challenging for openings and for change. This dynamic interaction is a vital part of community participation.

Action for change is usually stimulated by the contradictions that emerge from this interaction. There is not a finite point at which community participation will be achieved, it can never be a goal or target that is absolutely met and 'ticked off'. Community action for change is a dynamic process which evolves and develops in response to circumstances and situations. This is part of what makes it such an exciting process to be part of.

We hope the booklet conveys some of the energy and commitment that people in the UK at all levels are putting into the identification of health issues and needs, and into ways of developing strategies to meet these needs.

The UK National Health Service is just one small part of health support and provision – far more is happening in other settings than is ever realised or publicly acknowledged and we hope this publication will go some way in starting to make visible the vital contribution that community participation is making to health in the UK and wider world. Without community participation and involvement, 'Health for All' and the new Public Health will not be realised. It is a challenge for all of us involved or concerned to promote health to make participation a reality and not merely rhetoric.

Section 1: Keywords and Definitions

Keywords

Community concepts: a practical classification
Like all short definitions, the following will undoubtedly be debatable. The main aim is to provide definitions which will assist us to be consistent and hence make it easier to see the practical differences entailed in different approaches, whilst recognizing that action will often cross boundaries.

1. *Community:* people with a basis of common interest and network of personal interaction, grouped either on the basis of locality or on a specific shared concern or both.
2. *Community activity:* people doing things together or for each other with no stated form of organisation.
3. *Informal community care:* a type of community activity (2) directed to looking after others.
4. *Formal community care:* care provided by Authorities for people in their own homes. May seek to mobilise informal community care (3) as well.
5. *Self-help groups:* people grouping together in some form of local organisation effectively controlled by themselves for their own support in carrying out community activity (2) or informal community care (3).
6. *Groupwork:* a form of social work or other work using groups organised by an agency, unlike self-help groups (5) or the groups which carry out community action (7).
7. *Community action:* activity carried out by people under their own control in order to improve their collective conditions. May involve campaigning, negotiating with others, challenging authorities and power holders. May arise from or combine with self-help groups (5).
8. *Outreach:* action by authorities to deliver a service to those least likely to be getting proper benefit from it by taking it to the people in their own homes and social settings. May also seek to build links with community activity etc (1–5).
9. *Multidisciplinary work:* co-operation between professionals with different specialisations.
10. *Inter-agency work:* co-operation between services from the standpoint of their combined effects on particular communities, as seen by people in those communities.
11. *Social policy:* the policies of agencies with formal responsibilites for administering and providing services to society: government, local government, health authorities etc.
12. *Social work:* support to, or intervention in, the lives of individuals and families with particular problems.

13 *Community social work:* a form of social work which mobilises community activity (2) informal community care (3) or self-help groups (5).
14 *Community work:* stimulus and support for community action (7).
15 *Community development:* co-ordination of community work (14) with inter-agency work (10) and linking with social policy (11) especially with the intention of empowering a continually widening circle of participants.

In addition there are certain key terms which have an inbuilt ambiguity concerning how far they arise from a community, like community activity (2), informal community care (3), self-help groups (5) and community action (7), and how far they are provided for or willed upon a community by outside agencies, like formal community care (4), groupwork (6), outreach (8) and social policy (11).

In these cases we have to take care to indicate in a particular context whether we mean them in a strong sense (ie from within the community) or a weak sense (ie from outside the community).

16 *Community-based work:* either (a) work organised by a formal agency and placed within a community making use of outreach (8), inter-agency work (10), community social work (13) or community development (15) (weak sense) or (b) work organised by self-help groups (5) or community action (7) (strong sense).
17 *Community education:* either (a) non-vocational education, usually for adults (weak sense) or (b) education in skills relevant to community action and self-help (7 & 5) (strong sense).
18 *Community project:* either (a) programmes of work, organised by institutions for the improvement of conditions in a locality (weak sense) or (b) independent or quasi-independent local organisations dedicated to support for some combination of community activity (2) self-help (5) community action (7) or community development (15).

Source: Gabriel Chànàn – Community Projects Foundation
Prepared for forthcoming Health Education Authority publication R. Gorna, *Community Based AIDS Initiatives in the UK*, (soon to be available from Health Education Authority, England).

Definitions

The following definitions serve to expand on key aspects of communication and development and to provide a framework for the case studies which are included in Section 3.

The definitions and activities described are not mutually exclusive and all form part of the processes that are involved in this way of working in health promotion:

1 Formal participation

Citizens' participation in policy making, planning and/or implementation of decisions which relate to health, health promotion, the environment and care services.

The amount of participation can vary along a spectrum of low to high involvement as illustrated by the following chart:-

Degrees of participation
(From Brager and Specht, *Community Organising*, Columbia University Press, 1973, p. 39)

Degree	Participants' action	Illustrative mode
Low	None	The community is told nothing.
	Receives information	The organisation makes a plan and announces it. The community is convened for informational purposes; compliance is expected.
	Is consulted	The organisation tries to promote a plan and develop the support to facilitate acceptance of, or give sufficient sanction to, the plan so that administrative compliance can be expected.
	Advises	The organisation presents a plan and invites questions. It is prepared to modify the plan only if absolutely necessary.
	Plans jointly	The organisation presents a tentative plan subject to change and invites recommendations from those affected.
	Has delegated authority	The organisation identifies and presents a problem to the community; defines the limits and asks the community to make a series of decisions which can be embodied in a plan which it will accept.
High	Has control	The organisation asks the community to identify the problems and to make all the key decisions regarding goals and means. It is willing to help the community at each step accomplish its own goals, even to the extent of administrative control of the programme.

Participatory activities can include:
- Publicity about policies and decisions.
- Inviting comments, response to plans.
- Involving representatives on working groups, decision-making forums.
- Involving the community on management groups of projects, drawing up survey research methods.
- Setting up community health groups, forums and information centres which can act as a focus for participation.

2 Community action

Any activity or process undertaken by a community that involves action to obtain change. This may include:
- Pressure groups to exert influence (eg for a smoke-free environment).
- Self-care and self-reliance or mutual aid groups whereby people with a similar problem, condition or concern come together to share and gain support from others and to take responsibility for action around their own health.
- Voluntary bodies which contribute to assisting community action or undertaking it.
- Social movements – various forms of collective action by a group/community aimed at social change. In general, social movements are not institutionalised but arise from spontaneous social action directed at specific or widespread concerns, eg Community Health Movement.
- Advocacy projects/facilities which enable people who otherwise would not, to have a voice – eg via interpretation of people speaking on others' behalf.
- Lobbying local and national government.
- Direct action, eg challenging the practice of commercial and industrial bodies where they affect people's health or health potential.

3 Facilitating processes

Community organisation, enabling practices and related skills.

This aspect refers to activities which enable or facilitate processes whereby people in communities can enhance their support, skills, organisation, representation, range of influence and access to services.

This may include:
- Community analysis or surveys to understand and define communities' needs, in which the community is actively involved.
- Advocating change by producing written material, media work, training and negotiation.
- Organising specific project groups.
- Neighbourhood planning, de-centralising planning and management of services to local communities and encouraging and enabling their involvement.

- Maintaining momentum by, eg supporting groups and individuals.
- Developing people's skills.
- Network development and support.

4 Professional and community interface

Community development involves both people in communities, professionals who work with them and professionals/bureaucrats in positions of power. In order for the concerns and needs of communities to be realised, professionals and decision makers have to be open and able to respond.

The activities that aim to support the successful operation of such an interface will include:
- Training for community workers, professionals and decision makers, both separately and collectively.
- Reorientating professional roles and methods of working.
- Curriculum development to enable all professionals to be sensitive to community needs.
- Development of joint forums where communities and professionals can work together on equal terms.
- Development of other participation groups whereby communities can ultimately put their needs to professionals concerned.
- Management development to enable those with power and resources to be open to influence.
- Organisational development so that organisations and structures which will allow participation can evolve or be set up.

5 Strategic support

This concept relates to initiatives within organisations and policies which enable community action to develop, take place and be supported and disseminated. This can be at various levels, eg: national, regional or city, neighbourhood. Activities would include:
- Advocacy of theories, structures and strategies.
- Development and publication of materials.
- Funding.
- Advice and consultation.
- Network development and support.
- Training programmes.
- Forums/working parties.
- Research and evaluation.
- Making information available and accessible.

6 Definition of community development

We have included our working definition of community development in relation to health promotion in the hope that it will be a useful base for others to build on:

The basic aim of health promotion is to empower communities to own and control their own endeavours and destinies and to have direct involvement in the process of change.

Community development encompasses a commitment to a holistic approach to health which recognises the central importance of social support and social networks. A community development way of working attempts to facilitate individual and collective action around common needs and concerns which are identified by the community itself, rather than being imposed from outside.

This means that individuals and communities need to be fully involved in partnerships and networks to set priorities, make decisions, plan strategies and implement them in order to achieve better health.

To make this possible people need to be supported to come together. Both professional boundaries and statutory organisations need to be opened up, and flexible systems that rely on co-operative negotiated approaches need to be developed. For effective health promotion, public participation in all aspects of health is essential at all levels. This includes continuous access to information, learning opportunities, financial support and a real chance to influence decision making. Issues of openness, structure, equity and accessibility must be addressed as an integral part of a healthy public policy; and priority must be given to enabling the active involvement of people experiencing deprivation and powerlessness, in all aspects of health promotion and policy.

Within community development for health

'Community' can be defined geographically or as a community of interests eg: a street, a housing estate/neighbourhood, a women's group, a black group, a pensioners' group. People identify for themselves which communities they feel part of.

More stress is placed on issues common to many members of a community rather than concentrating upon individuals.

Community work prioritises activity with deprived groups and issues related to inequalities in health.

Problems and concerns are seen to be interlinked and not compartmentalised into employment, housing, health, education etc. Thus a community development approach to health promotion encompasses all aspects of people's lives that relate to their social, mental and physical well-being and potential.

There is a recognition of social, economic and environmental influences on health which are often outside the individual's control.

The process of working together for health is seen as important in itself as well as any outcome it might achieve. The main emphasis in community development is action and change.

An overall or holistic view of health is taken rather than concentrating on parts of the body, diseases, symptoms or particular issues.

There is encouragement to value people whatever their background, capabilities, sex, race, sexual orientation etc, and an attempt to actively counter prejudice and discrimination wherever it occurs.

It is fitting that any definition will evolve and change over the next few years, as theory, practice and networking develop.

Section 2: Case Studies

Introduction to case studies

The case studies in this section illustrate different aspects of community action in health. They are divided into categories using a system suggested by the World Health Organisation and the Health Education Authority in England (definitions of these categories are included in the previous section) i.e.
- Formal participation – in decision-making mechanisms
- Community action – community level activities & mechanisms
- Facilitating processes – enabling within the community
- Professional and community interface
- Strategic support.

Within each category each case study describes *one* aspect of the work of a project by looking at its main features, the background to that piece of work, information on how the community is involved or represented in that work and who they are, examples of success in this area and lessons to be learnt.

Inevitably this focus on just one aspect of a project's work leaves out other aspects which in practice interweave to give a coherent whole. The wide range of case studies illustrates the breadth of community participation in health. This shows that complementary work is needed at all levels to build a holistic strategy for the advancement of public health.

Formal participation

Title of Project/Work: **Community Care Project (CCP), National Council for Voluntary Organisations (NCVO)**
Source of Material: NCVO Community Care Project *The Work of the National Unit 1984–1988*
Further Information: Community Care Project, NCVO, 26 Bedford Square, London WC1B 3HU
Telephone 071-636 4066

Main features considered here: Formal participation in the 'Progress In Partnership' Working Party set up by the Government Department of Health and Social Security. This was through the giving of evidence and advice to the Working Party via the Joint Planning Working Group of Voluntary Organisations set up by the Community Care Project.
Background: The CCP was set up by NCVO in 1984 in response to the growing demand for community care services, a lack of voluntary sector participation in the statutory planning of such services, and the need for good practice in voluntary/statutory relationships. Involvement in the Working Party was seen as one method of achieving this.

Representation: Voluntary organisations concerned with the client groups most affected, relevant national agencies and people from the local voluntary sector involved in joint planning are represented on the Joint Planning Working Group of Voluntary Organisations.

Examples: Through this participation the voluntary sector have made recommendations to Government on increasing user and voluntary sector participation in planning, commented on other relevant Government papers and liaised with them over particular local difficulties.

Lessons: In order to have an effective voice on the Working Party, considerable work was required to bring together voluntary organisations to share information, agree objectives and put forward clear proposals, to ensure a strong link between local action and national policy.

Title of Project/Work: **Brent Sickle Cell + Thalassaemia Centre**
Source of Material: Elizabeth N. Anionwu *Community Development Approaches to Sickle Cell Anaemia* 1988 and *Running a Sickle Cell Centre: Community Counselling* 1988
Further Information: Brent Sickle Cell + Thalassaemia Centre, Willesden Hospital, Harlesden Road, London NW10 3RY
Telephone 081-459 1292

Main features considered here: Formal participation by the community in the development of services within the National Health Service (NHS) for sickle cell anaemia. This was through the establishment of specialist community groups, such as the Sickle Cell Society and the creation of counselling and screening services within the NHS.

Background: The processes described grew out of criticism of the NHS for failing to provide adequate services. There was collaboration between community pressure groups and some, particularly black, health workers within the NHS.

Representation: Local health workers, patients and parents were initially involved in pressing for change which lead to the establishment of the local self-help group in 1977. Out of this grew the national Sickle Cell Society which, informed by visits to existing centres in the United States of America, was instrumental in the establishment of the Brent Sickle Cell Centre within the NHS.

Examples: Through the use of community networks, black and local media, sending information to health workers and visits to patients and their families, the numbers of people using the Centre each year for information, blood tests and counselling has risen from 180 in 1980 to 800 in 1988. Over 50% are now self-referrals.

Lessons: The close initial working together of the Sickle Cell Society, a national charity, and the Sickle Cell Centre, based within the NHS, was crucial to the success of the project.

Title of Project/Work: **Voluntary and Community Sector Forum for Joint Planning in Hackney (FJP)**
Source of Material: Job Description of Voluntary Sector Co-ordinator (Joint Planning); Work Programme; etc; all 1989
Further Information: FJP, Hackney Community Action, 90 De Beauvoir Road, London N1 4EN
Telephone 071-923 1962

Main features considered here: The work of the Voluntary Sector Co-ordinator in enabling the formal involvement of the FJP in advising the District Health Authority (DHA) and Local Authority (LA) on Joint Planning issues.
Background: The successful application for joint funding from the DHA and LA for a post to develop the FJP was a recognition that the Joint Planning system was geared towards the needs of the statutory sector. Greater co-ordination and participation by community groups was seen as necessary for the protection of services and the development of better integrated services.
Representation: The FJP feeds into the DHA's Integrated Project Groups (IPGs) where the community and voluntary sector is represented by umbrella organisations, user groups or specific groups. The representatives are nominated by their various organisations at the request of the Joint Planning Office. The FJP is seeking to address the fact that disadvantaged groups are underpresented within the Joint Planning structures and thus within the FJP.
Examples: The worker aims to involve more community IPG representatives in the FJP, particularly from black and ethnic minority groups, improve their accountability to the wider community sector and ensure the FJP takes up policy issues. This is through developmental outreach work (to community groups), developing the FJP's structure (eg. accountability), developing an infrastructure (eg. training) and policy work.
Lessons: All aspects of the strategy are developed together and feed into each other. Increased local participation is seen as important as effective policy work.

Title of Project/Work: **Salford Community Health Project (SCHP)**
Source of Material: Information from Project Worker
Further Information: SCHP, Higher Broughton Health Centre, Bevendon Square, Salford M7 0UF
Telephone 061 792 6969.

Main features considered here: An integral feature of SCHP is developing new and using existing mechanisms for promoting community participation in health decisions, eg supporting members of community groups to stand for election to the Community Health Council (CHC), to sit on the formal management committee of the Project, or to participate in the Women's Education Forum which is formally recognized by the Education Committee of the Local Authority.

Background: This work was a natural development from neighbourhood-based work which resulted in a number of different issues being recognised as needing change in policies at local and national level. The community then identified ongoing participation in decision making as a means to achieving these changes and ensuring that services become more responsive.

Representation: Community members of the CHC are elected from a range of voluntary and community health groups. Members of the SCHP management committee are elected at the AGM from projects supported by SCHP. Members of the Women's Education Forum are self-selected from community health groups.

Examples: The Women's Education Forum has successfully campaigned for a policy on women's education. It is now a very active force in the Joint Working Group which is drawing up the policy as well as continuing to support a range of women's education courses in local areas.

Lessons: It is hard work as very few of the formal mechanisms for participation in health decision making are accessible to people in local communities. This actively mitigates against the active involvement of more than one or two people so only a very limited number of people can be directly involved. This has forced the development of new structures and mechanisms which are more all-encompassing.

Title of Project/Work: **Wirral Womens Health Network (WWHN)**
Sources of Material: WWHN *Women Influencing Decision-Making Structures* 1989
Further Information: WWHN, c/o Well Women Centre, St. Catherine's Hospital, Birkenhead, Wirral, Merseyside
Telephone 051 6785111 × 3514

Main features considered here: The formal participation of women through the WWHP in the Women and Health Tripartite Group (WHTG) with senior officers from the Health Authority and the Social Services Department. This group was formed to build an overall policy across the borough on women's health initiatives. It is now in the process of becoming the Women's Health Policy and Planning Group linked to the decision-making processes of the Joint Consultative Committee, which will enable the WWHN to have a voice within the established structure.

Background: Following the establishment of an extremely successful Well Women Clinic session in the area and the continuous development of women's health courses and self-help groups across the borough by a part-time community health worker, the WWHN was set up. It was formed as an advisory group for this worker and as an umbrella organisation. A local councillor became interested in this group which led to the establishment of the WHTG (as above).

Representation: The WWHN was formed from local women's health groups, the Well Women centre, voluntary workers, community organisations and individual women who showed an interest in health issues. They aimed to comprise at least half of the WHTG.

Examples: The WWHN developed the following set of principles for meetings of the WHTG: setting the agenda themselves, meeting in an accessible place, convenient timing, equal numbers with statutory representatives, preparing a policy document quoting 'Health for All' principles for support, pre-meeting, supporting each other, taking minutes.

Lessons: The women found that the strengths they had built up through their women and health, assertiveness and counselling courses could be used to influence power structures such as WHTG.

Title of Project/Work: **Healthy Sheffield 2000 (HS2000)**
Source of Material: Improving the Health of Sheffield People and *HS 2000 Organisational Structure,* HS2000, 1989
Further Information: HS 2000, Town Hall Chambers, 1 Barker's Pool, Sheffield S1 1EN
Telephone 0742 734645

Main features considered here: Formal participation of the community in HS2000 through formal representation on the HS2000 planning team, subcommittees and working groups which feed into Sheffield's Joint Consultative Committee. Also there is regular formal consultation at all significant stages and open structures for communication from community interests and open access to information at all levels.

Background: HS2000 was a response to health inequality in Sheffield and a collective concern by the City Council, Health Authority and voluntary sector to respond to the challenge of reducing health inequality whilst improving the health of the whole population. It aims to be an initiative which encourages all organisations in the city to be more aware of the health impact of their policies and services.

Representation: Community involvement is diverse. Formal representation on the HS2000 committees is from the Council of Voluntary Service, the Council for Community Relations and the Community Health Council, who in turn represent community concerns. There is informal involvement from many community interests through the Community Health Network which is practically supported by HS2000 staff and through direct contact with some local groups.

Examples: HS2000 has provided support for the Community Health Network which provides a forum for those interested in community health development. It has also helped to facilitate the formation of the Women's

Health Forum and the Black Health Forum.
Lessons: The work has shown that participatory ways of working take time and so there is a need to use a flexible approach and not set unrealistic timescales. Similarly formal relationships need to be supported with good informal contacts and joint working.

Title of Project/Work: **Ethnic Minorities Health Care Forum**
Source of Material: Information from Project Worker
Further Information: Ethnic Minorities Health Care Forum, 441 Harrow Road, London W10
Telephone 081-960 5746

Main features considered here: The Forum is a voluntary body. It aims to bring to the attention of local voluntary and statutory organisations the issues concerning the health services that black and ethnic minority people receive and to press for change. In 1987 it was asked by the Health Authority to provide some input to their senior management group on health and race issues. Participation was withdrawn, however, because it was felt the Health Authority were not considering the issues within the context of an Equal Opportunities Policy.
Background: The Forum was formed after a one-day workshop on black and ethnic minority health which was organised by the then Health Education Council, as those attending felt that a more permanent basis was needed for the work. The District had a high proportion of people from black and ethnic minority backgrounds and over 100 different languages are spoken in the area.
Representation: The Forum do not formally represent anyone as there are no elections, but those involved include Afro-Caribbean, Spanish, Portuguese, Bengali and Chinese people.
Examples: The District Health Authority have since appointed an Equal Opportunities Officer with whom the Forum have liaised. It has also advertised for a Health and Race Officer at senior level and the Forum have met with the responsible manager to advise on the job description and advertising and discuss what they can offer the post. Also the Forum has worked through the Family Practitioner Committee to successfully halt the internal immigration controls that were operating in some health offices.
Lessons: Participation is difficult, both because Forum members are already overloaded in their work and because the Health Authority lacks credibility, closing essential services which the Forum protested against, leaving the feeling that the Authority is not responsive.

Community action

Title of Project/Work: **National Community Health Resource (NCHR)**
Source of Material: NCHR Report *A New Voice for Health* 1988; NCHR Agenda for Annual General Meeting 1988

Further information: NCHR, 15 Britannia Street, London WC1X 9JP
Telephone 071-837 2426

Main features considered here: Co-ordination of the Community Health Movement in Britain as an example of a social movement. Also developing networks, advice and information, training and education, organising conferences and seminars.

Background: NCHR was formed in 1988 through the amalgamation of two similar organisations, with a brief to support and promote community health activity. In turn this grew out of the need to support community development for health at frontline level and help the movement to 'find a voice' following the growth in community health initiatives in the 1970s.

Involvement: NCHR is a representative body for the community health movement with membership drawn from people directly involved with community health initiatives in the voluntary and statutory sectors and other workers, policy makers and researchers with an interest in community health. Initially the membership of women and black people was especially encouraged.

Examples: In 1987 the Women's Health Network was established after the national 'Better Health for Women' conference in Harlow. This continues to co-ordinate women's health initiatives and develop new ones, and ran the women's conference 'Feeling Strong, Growing Stronger' in 1989.

Lessons: It has been essential for the successful co-ordination and development of the community health movement that NCHR works along community development lines. It operates at many levels; the local/regional/national, and the grassroots/infrastructure/policy. This is also reflected in the way it involves its members and in its decision-making structures.

Title of Project/Work: **Brent Health Emergency (BHE)**
Source of Material: Brent Community Health Council (CHC) *Annual Report* 1984
Further Information: Brent Community Health Council, 16 High Street, London NW10
Telephone 081-961 2028

Main features considered here: Acting as a pressure group to press Brent Council and the District Health Authority to defend Brent's health services and support the struggle for decent health care. (NB. Although the events described here have now passed, it is included because it is a well documented campaign with useful lessons to be learnt.)

Background: The BHE was formed in 1984 in response to the need to form a broad-based and campaigning organisation outside of the CHC structure to defend health services in Brent. The group wanted to highlight the lack of democracy within the National Health Service and the pressure on the

District Health Authority through threats of dismissal from the Region, to implement cuts in services.

Involvement: The BHE involved local people, health unions, community groups, borough Councillors (elected Members of Local Government) and the CHC.

Examples: BHE organised a 'health festival' to draw in more people from all sections of the community and provide information on health cuts, services and alternatives in an accessible way. This was followed later by a rally of 500 people to mobilise support and lobby, with a mass attendance at a District Health Authority meeting followed by a number of local meetings.

Lessons: Raising and utilising such a high level of community interest in health as an issue was enabled through a high profile campaign and the imaginative attempts to involve people. It was felt that the involvement of the trade unions, the financial support offered by Brent Council (Local Authority) and the backup from the CHC were necessary to maintain momentum.

Title of Project/Work: **Health in Retirement – Fulham North**
Source of Material: Information from Project Worker
Further Information: Health In Retirement, Bishop Creighton House Settlement, 378 Lillie Road, London SW6 7PH
Telephone 071-385 6295

Main features considered here: The project encourages community action through the setting up of community health groups. Pensioners are involved from the beginning in planning the group, setting the programme and eventually self-managing the group. Examples include the Older Women's Group, the Older Men's Group, estate-based Older Pensioner Groups, the Black Senior Citizens Health Group and the Sleep Group.

Background: While the earlier 'Activity In Retirement' project was coming to a close, it became apparent to the worker that there was a need for a pensioners' health project to ease social isolation and encourage mental and physical stimulation. There was also a strong need to tackle ageism in all aspects of health.

Involvement: Almost all the pensioners involved are from the Fulham North area and are working class. Most are women. They are also involved in the working party for the Well Pensioner Project (see below) along with paid workers from different agencies.

Examples: Contact with pensioners in the health groups and the ageism in the health service that this revealed, led the project to set up a working party with the aim of establishing a Well Pensioners Project which would provide a shop front for pensioners to drop in for physical health check-ups, use the café and the counselling service. It would be non-institutional with

pensioners trained to do much of the work, especially outreach. Funding is currently being sought.
Lessons: The project's sole worker has found it important to involve workers from other agencies, to provide the work with more continuity as well as to spread the message to other organisations and prevent isolation. The big challenge has been in combatting ageism.

Title of Project/Work: **Women's Health Information and Support Centre, Northampton**
Source of Material: Information from Project Worker
Further Information: Women's Health Information and Support Centre, Junction 7, Hazelwood Road, Northampton NN1 1LG
Telephone 0604 39723

Main features considered here: Volunteer provision of a two-day drop in service for women, which includes health information, pregnancy testing and someone to talk to. In addition education courses are run for women.
Background: The Centre began in 1984 as a project of the Unemployment Centre in Northampton, with the help of a paid worker, as a response to the needs of local women which were not being met by statutory services. It became independent the following year when it continued with voluntary staff. It has received three years funding from the Government via the 'Opportunities For Volunteering' Programme and has a small ongoing grant from the Health Authority.
Involvement: All those involved are volunteers who have responded to a recruiting drive or word of mouth contact. All volunteers attend a women's health listening skills training course, unsuitable volunteers being redirected through this process. The project is managed through both a volunteers' committee and a management committee.
Examples: These consist of the drop-in service and education courses for women mentioned above.
Lessons: The project would have preferred a stricter selection process for choosing volunteers, had there been more than enough volunteers to choose from, which has not been the case since 1985.

Title of Project/Work: **Bradford Action on Health**
Source of Material: Information from Health Education Authority (HEA)
Further Information: Bradford Action on Health, c/o Community Projects Foundation (CPF) North, 20 Central Road, Leeds
Telephone 0532 460909

Main features considered here: The project uses a community development approach to health education in Bradford with a particular emphasis on HIV and AIDS. They began with a developmental phase, linking to and working with existing networks and organisations, to work out how best to structure and plan the second operational phase. They concentrate on working with the community in ways that are acceptable to different cultures and traditions.

Background: CPF had been funded by the HEA to produce a literature and network search on 'Community Based AIDS Initiatives' (forthcoming). Following that, together with the District Health Authority they obtained funds from the HEA to run the project. The work will be intensively evaluated.

Involvement: The project seeks to work particularly with Asian and ethnic minority groups. The Community Health Forum, Community Health Council, Ethnic Minority Health Forum and the Community Relations Council are all involved.

Examples: The operational phase is likely to have two strands, outreach work and a drop-in centre. This will be more like a community health centre, based in the city centre, offering advice and information and activities for a range of different groups eg. youth groups, pensioners' groups and women's groups.

Lessons: The work shows that HIV and AIDS need to be part of a wider approach to community health and sexuality issues. A crucial practical lesson is the necessity of employing a worker who speaks the language of the target community.

Title of Project/Work: **Self-Help Action Project, Herefordshire**
Source of Material: Information from Project Workers; Final Report of Project 1989
Further Information: Self-Help Unit, 25 Castle Street, Hereford HR12 NU Telephone 0432 263757

Main features considered here: A three-year project aimed at supporting self-help groups in the area through providing practical help (contacts, publicity, information etc), networking, co-working, dissemination of the self-help philosophy to the general public, creating opportunities for people to come together for mutual support (sometimes through adult education classes) and responding to individuals who express an interest. This is within the general aim of using self-help to build confidence, tackle stress and aid communication.

Background: This is one of the eighteen projects set up on an experimental pilot three-year basis by the Department of Health and Social Security and managed centrally through the Self-Help Alliance, a national voluntary organisation.

Involvement: The Project works with around ninety self-help groups in Herefordshire, covering a wide range of health and welfare issues. There is particular emphasis on carers groups (usually friends or relatives caring for others, usually disabled or infirm, in their homes).

Examples: The Project was approached by an individual in need of support and with her, set up a 'What Next?' group for people with mental health problems. This began as an adult education class, with the co-operation of the local branch of MIND, (a mental health organisation).

Lessons: In Herefordshire it has been important not just to see self-help in terms of groups, but as also applying to individuals through the concept of self-care. Much of the work of the Project has been on a one-to-one basis with individuals. When a group is required, it has been helpful to start it with an adult education class on the topic, in co-operation with the local branch of the Workers Educational Association, which may then evolve into a group.

Title of Project/Work; **Granton Health Project: Pilton Food Co-op**
Source of Material: Information from Project Worker
Further Information: Granton Health Project, 3 West Pilton Park, Edinburgh EH4 4EC, Scotland
Telephone 031 332 0871

Main features considered here: Organising a voluntary food co-operative which is mainly run by women on a weekly basis. The van goes to the wholesale market and buys food in bulk. Local club members (about 100 at present) come and buy in smaller quantities. Small amounts of food are packed up for local pensioner clubs and sold there also.

Background: The Health Project already worked with a food co-op for pensioners. They started work in a new area where there was high unemployment and low incomes. Food in the local small shops, especially fruit and vegetables, was expensive and of poor quality. The project wanted to respond in very practical ways and local residents, with the help of the Project decided to organise collective food shopping for themselves.

Involvement: There are about 100 members of the food co-op from the local area. Of these about ten are active (all women apart from the male driver) meeting monthly with the Project. A crèche worker looks after their children while they are on co-op business.

Examples: The co-op has expanded their sale of wholefoods. Other food co-ops have since set up in other parts of Edinburgh.

Lessons: The food co-op group has needed regular backup from community workers at the project, usually at the monthly business meetings, to help with problems, disagreements and upsets. Help in the cash management of large sums of money is also important. Many members have grown in confidence and skill eg working out prices and dealing with complaints. The co-op is now looking into starting a community business venture.

Facilitating processes

Title of Project/Work: **Wells Park Health Project**
Source of Material: Wells Park Health Project *Annual Report 1986/87;*

Notes on Review and Planning Day 1988; Newsletter 1989
Further Information: Wells Park Health Project, 1A Wells Park Road, London SE26 6JE
Telephone 081-291 3322

Main features considered here: Maintaining the momentum of community input, interest and energy in community groups and organisations.

Background: Wells Park Health Project was set up in 1983 as a response to the need for a community development approach to health and through the joint initiative of a community worker and a general practitioner. It operated from a community development approach from the beginning, aiming to enable local people to meet together and take action to change anything in the local area which prevents people from being healthy.

Involvement: Currently the main users of the Health Project from the community are women with children, women over fifty, carers, diabetics, and the mentally ill. The role of the Project in maintaining community momentum is to encourage local people to come together and to facilitate their active participation.

Examples: The community development worker spent some time in supporting a local man in doing the groundwork to set up a carers' self help group and then in helping the group to work out how it wanted to develop and maintain itself. This included visits to people's homes as well as regular attendance at the group.

Lessons: The worker needed to maintain a balance between supporting individuals in groups and helping the group to develop a support structure of its own.

Title of Project/Work: **Alzheimer's Disease Society (ADS)**
Source of Material: Alzheimer's Disease Society, *Annual Report 1987/88* and Newsletters
Further Information: Alzheimer's Disease Society, 158–160 Balham High Road, London SW12 9BN
Telephone 081-675 6557/8/9/0

Main features considered here: Facilitating the process of developing skills for carers looking after those with, and coping with, a chronic illness. Its aims are to give support to families by linking them with each other through a monthly newsletter, regular provision of information, publications and support services and through guidance to local branches and groups. The ADS also provides information, education and training to promote research on the disease and press for the provision of adequate services for those coping with it.

Background: The ADS was established in 1979 by a carer in response to the need to support others caring for those with the disease.

Involvement: All carers of people with Alzheimer's Disease can become

members. The Society was aiming for a total membership of 10,000 in 1988/9.
Examples: The Society has helped promote daycare in Middlesbrough so that carers can have a break; a sitting service in Salisbury for the same purpose; and a newsletter for members with a questions and answers page on issues related to the disease, practical tips for carers, information and advice, and examples of good practice in this area by voluntary and statutory organisations.
Lessons: The ADS through its work has seen the need to build partnerships with relevant organisations and so it has begun to encourage links with the Carers' National Association, Age Concern and the Centre for Policy on Ageing, in order to focus more effectively on the needs of people with the disease.

Title of Project/Work: **Community Health Surveys**
Source of Material: Sue Blennerhasset, *A Review of Community Health Surveys*, National Community Health Resource (NCHR)
Further Information: NCHR Information, 15 Britannia Street, London WC1X 9JP
Telephone 071-837 2426

Main features considered here: Use of community health surveys as a method of analysing the community to facilitate the design of successful health promotion programmes. Such surveys are carried out by a wide variety of agencies from the voluntary and statutory sectors, ranging from community groups to academic institutions. They therefore operate from within different frameworks eg. community development, health promotion, or community medicine. They tend to use different methods according to the framework eg. postal questionnaires and telephone surveys (health promotion) or in-depth interviews and door-to-door visiting (community development).
Background: Currently Health Education/Promotion Units (locally-based centres within Health Authorities) tend to carry out surveys to create a 'baseline' from which to evaluate health programmes, while Community Health Projects tend to use them to find out about the concerns and needs of local people.
Involvement: According to the framework used, the involvement of the community from the catchment area may be limited to 'being surveyed' or extended to planning and carrying it out.
Examples: Successful results for Health Education Units include better informed health workers. For Community Health Projects they include showing the need for improved services, such as well-women sessions at clinics, through mounting a campaign or informing planners.

Lessons: For the community, surveys are not always the best method of getting the information needed – they can be time-consuming, create suspicion or seem like stating the obvious. The advantages are increased knowledge, generating enthusiasm, setting up new groups. The community will learn more from the survey if they are involved from the very beginning.

Title of Project/Work: **The Buddy Group**
Source of Material: The Trust Newsletter, Number 5, July 1989
Further Information: The Buddy Group, The Terrence Higgins Trust (THT), 52–54 Gray's Inn Road, London WC1X 8JU
Telephone 071-831 0330

Main features considered here: Facilitating a community support structure for people with AIDS through the use of a co-ordinated system of volunteers or buddies. On joining, buddies make a commitment both to a person with AIDS and to a local group, where they give and receive support through regular, obligatory support group meetings. These meetings are co-ordinated through an Area Co-ordinator who also ensures they are a vehicle of communication between buddies and the THT in general.
Background: The Buddy Group was set up by the THT in response to the need to provide intensive one-to-one support to people with AIDS. There are currently 195 buddies divided into ten areas of Greater London.
Involvement: Volunteer buddies are drawn from all sections of the community in order to try to offer the person with AIDS a choice in terms of age, gender and sexuality. They are approached through a series of recruitment campaigns.
Examples: Selection of interested volunteers is through an initial interview with the Volunteer Co-ordinator, followed by an intensive training day at THT and an in-depth interview which includes questions about their motivation and how they see the buddying relationship fitting in to their existing commitments. If accepted they start to attend local support meetings and the next available residential training course before visiting a person with AIDS.
Lessons: It was felt that the residential training courses for buddies should not be part of the assessment of volunteers, so that they could provide a safer environment in which volunteers could share their apprehensions about the prospect of befriending someone with AIDS.

Title of Project/Work: **Women's Health and Information Support Centre (WHISC) Ltd, Liverpool**
Source of Material: Information from Project Worker
Further Information: WHISC, 104 Bold Street, Liverpool L1 4RY
Telephone 051 709 1938

Main features considered here: Facilitating the development of self-help women's health groups and of volunteer workers for the WHISC drop-in, which in turn facilitates a constantly developing women's health network in Liverpool, through the provision of a two-year part-time training course in Women's Health.

Background: The two-year course evolved from a smaller venture which began in 1985. By that time, WHISC had been set up on an unfunded basis as part of the Community Education Project in the area. They wanted to run a drop-in for women and felt training would put this on a sound footing and enable expertise from all over Liverpool to be gained.

Involvement: Women attend the courses from all over Liverpool, whether they are interested in their own health and development, want to set up self-help groups, or become involved in WHISC.

Examples: Women from the Weller Street Housing Co-op who had been on their own women's health course, then went onto WHISC's and became WHISC volunteers, bringing in their own expertise. Other women have used the course to encourage them to go into further education. The course has had an effect on the 'Healthy Cities' network by arranging an exchange with women from Belfast 'Healthy City'.

Lessons: Training provided an important organisational element for WHISC, helping it to carry on while still unfunded. However, it was felt that even if WHISC had not been given funding, the training would have an immediate application for personal growth and development. An important philosophy for the training has been the view that all women attending the course themselves have the potential to train, so that the traditional distance between tutor and student is gradually broken down.

Title of Project/Work: **Salford Community Health Project (SCHP) Crèche Awareness Group**
Source of Material: Information from Project Worker
Further Information: Crèche Awareness Group, SCHP, Higher Broughton Health Centre, Bevendon Square, Salford M7 0UF
Telephone 061 792 6969

Main features considered here: Developing a campaign on crèche provision based on the principle of redressing inequalities and facilitating women's access to services, work and leisure. The campaign produced a Crèche Report accepted by the local authority, information on crèches and worked with a number of agencies and groups, in particular the Crèche Co-op, the Women's Health Forum, the Women's Education Forum and the Women's Centre, to develop innovatory and practical crèche services.

Background: Originally, the SCHP ran a number of 'voluntary' crèches alongside its women's health courses which led to the setting up of the Crèche Project, now the Crèche Co-op. They worked with a Crèche Group,

part of a citywide Women's Network, to develop the campaigning Crèche Awareness Group as above.
Involvement: Self-selected members of women's health groups throughout the city are involved plus a local councillor.
Examples: The acceptance of the Salford Crèche Report at District Labour Party led to a greater commitment to develop crèche facilities in the city and a grant of £500 from the Community Chest to develop the campaign.
Lessons: The campaign was very much geared to involving women Councillors jointly in its activities so that they developed an awareness of the need for crèches and much anti-feminist bias was broken down. This also meant that local women involved learnt a lot about power structures.

Title of Project/Work: **Inner City Mental Health Project, Bristol**
Source of Material: Project Report and Evaluation, 1989
Further Information: Inner City Mental Health Project, The Manse, Parkway Methodist Church, Conduit Place, St. Werburghs, Bristol BS2 9RU Telephone 0272 556098

Main features considered here: Creating accessible, 'user friendly', culturally sensitive and anti-racist mental health services for hard-to-reach groups in the inner city. The Project provides group work in hostels, day centres, hospitals and community halls, and counselling for individuals and their families in their homes. It offers support on racial harassment.
Background: Research in Bristol by the University showed disturbing levels of mental ill health among the homeless and minority ethnic groups, with a health service that was insensitive to their needs and inaccessible to and alienated from the community. It was also found that Afro-Caribbeans were often detained by the police and put into psychiatric care by the police and more likely to have compulsory treatment and that Asians rarely used the services.
Involvement: Users, survivors, relatives, professional and informal carers, local Black groups and self-help groups are all directly involved in the Project and are members of the consultative group along with the local Council for Community Relations. The local churches are involved through the use of their premises.
Examples: A Black Self-Help Survivors Group for people of African origin was set up by the Project and has since become a self-help organisation.
Lessons: Work to empower people to redefine their needs has put pressure on service providers. Community action facilitated by ongoing consultation and involvement has helped local people generate their own resources and gain access to mechanisms for participation. Multi-racial teamwork with a commitment to challenging racism has been necessary to work creatively within a health service without a conscious equal opportunity and anti-racist strategy.

Title of Project/Work: **Community Service Volunteers (CSV) Young Peoples HIV/AIDS Media Project**
Source of Material: Information from Project Worker
Further Information: CSV Volunteer Programme, 237 Pentonville Road, London N1 9NJ
Telephone 071-278 6601

Main features considered here: Using young people as volunteers to facilitate the spread of information, by various means including the media and local radio, among their peers, on how to protect themselves from HIV and AIDS. The aim is to help prevent the spread of HIV and AIDS among the under twenty five age group.
Background: CSV had a great deal of experience of the power of young people as volunteers to influence and effect change. CSV were concerned about the general spread of AIDS and HIV infection, and felt there was a need for pilot projects to test out new approaches in educating and informing young people about this as there was no tried and tested successful model.
Involvement: The Project have decided to recruit volunteers via local radio initially, and then explore other methods of recruitment. As CSV has a non-rejection policy, all volunteers coming forward will be used, according to their particular skills. The volunteers will be formed into a Youth Action Group and direct the Project for themselves with specialist help as needed and as guided by the Project Leader, for example from Health Education Officers, the Youth Service and Trainers.
Examples: The Project is only just beginning to get off the ground. However, CSV has twenty seven years of experience of using volunteers in situations of human need and each year about 2,000 volunteers work in face to face settings with people.
Lessons: It is too soon to say.

Title of Project/Work: **Keighley Tranx Project**
Source of Material: Information from Project Worker and Case Studies
Further Information: Keighley Tranx Project, Temple Row Centre, Keighley, West Yorkshire
Telephone 0535 604119

Main features considered here: Confidential advisory service for individuals who wish to withdraw from the use of tranquillisers through individual appointments and introductions to groups. The service is advertised through the newspaper, radio phone-ins, notices, talks and open days.
Background: The Project identified the need for a different approach from prescribing tranquillisers for the health problems that women experience. They felt that women need a great deal of support and advice to withdraw from tranquillisers that they may have taken for many years and to deal with

the original problem that tranquillisers were prescribed for.
Involvement: The main involvement is from non-professional women who have suffered and overcome the problem and wish to help prevent others suffering as they have done. Counselling courses are organised for them and some have gone on to set up self-help groups eg. Tranquilliser Withdrawal Support Group, Stillbirth Group, Cot Death Group, Mastectomy Support Group, Walking Group, Swimming Group.
Examples: The Project is in the process of setting up a 'Senior Health Awareness Project' with the help of three local nurses, which will be for and run by the over fifties to help overcome the shame felt by people on tranquillisers which discourages their seeking help.
Lessons: A 24-hour telephone support service was seen as essential to the success of the Project. The availability of this sort of support as well as help in dealing with the original health problem was seen as important as counselling in achieving success.

Title of Project/Work: **Research Project on Assertiveness and Women's Health Education**
Source of Material: Chrissie Whitehead *Assertiveness and Women's Health Education*, Health Education Authority (HEA), 1989
Further Information: Professional and Community Development Division, Health Education Authority, Hamilton House, Mabledon Place, London WC1
Telephone 071-383 3833

Main features considered here: Production of a report as a process facilitating the learning from and use of assertiveness training within women's health education achieved by sending questionnaires to a large range of organisations, interviewing individuals and running group seminars. It is planned that it will lead to the production of a related training pack.
Background: The HEA felt there was little information available on the level of existing provision and resources for assertiveness training within women's health and so decided to commission a research project to fill this gap.
Involvement: A large number of organisations were sent questionnaires but those interviewed and attending group seminars were based on recommendations at local level within Cambridge and Liverpool for their work with women on assertiveness.
Examples: As part of the research a session was held in Liverpool for those who train women in assertiveness. As a spin-off, the women have felt positive and validated about the work they do and continued to meet as a support group, sharing ideas and resources and intend to write and publish their own assertiveness training materials.

Lessons: The report was useful in providing a number of spin-offs in addition to its original aims because information was obtained through the community action process of relationship building and tapping into networks. Care was taken to feedback all the information compiled.

Professional and community interface

Title of Project/Work: **National Community Health Resource (NCHR) Training Project**
Source of Material: NCHR Training Project Steering Group
Training Policy Strategy 1989 and *Terms of Reference 1989*
Further Information: NCHR Training Project, 15 Britannia Street, London WC1X 9JP
Telephone 071-837 2426

Main features considered here: Use of the Training Project to facilitate a two-way learning process between health and community professionals. Its aims include offering a series of training courses to community health workers which would in turn enable them to train others, and to support the regional training networks.
Background: The Training Project was set up in 1988 out of the training work in community development and health carried out by NCHR. It is funded by the Health Education Authority.
Involvement: The main audience for the Training Project is community health professionals who use a community development approach to health. They include community development workers and community-based health professionals. This interface takes place at local, regional and national level through the training courses and infrastructure built up by the Project.
Examples: The Project managed the training of a core of facilitators for the National Community Health Conference in Newcastle in 1989. Community activists, community development workers and health professionals were trained together to develop similar skills and exchange existing skills.
Lessons: The interface is more productive when there is a shared definition of a 'community development approach to health'. This had been facilitated by the earlier work of NCHR and by the way the Training Project operates at various levels, local, regional and national.

Title of Project/Work: **Health Visitor – Minority Ethnic Groups**
Source of Material: Information from Health Visitor (HV)
Further Information: Health Promotion Department, Green Lodge, Barratts Green Road, London NW10 7AP
Telephone 081-965 6566

Main features considered here: Liaison by the District Health Authority with community groups and organisations from the minority ethnic communities with the aim of developing health promotion work, usually in the form of health courses or health days. Current work is with the Arabic speaking community in collaboration with the Adult Education Institute.

Background: The post was created through one of the recommendations of a project on ways in which the practice of HVs can be more community development orientated. One year into the project, the post was changed from one of working with community groups to working with ethnic minority groups which more accurately reflected current needs.

Involvement: The Health Visitor works alongside voluntary organisations such as the Migrants Unit and Moroccan Women's Project and statutory organisations like the 'English as a Second Language Department' of the Adult Education Institute, who are in direct contact with ethnic minority communities.

Examples: Looking with community groups at the available literature in Arabic on health services, has led to a clear demand for an updated and more locally relevant version, which will be worked on presently.

Lessons: Working in this way has created greater access to ways of assessing needs. However, it needs time to develop and reveals wide gaps in understanding the different ways of working between the voluntary sector and the National Health Service.

Title of Project/Work: **Community Development (CD) Curriculum in Health Education Training**
Source of Material: CD Group *Course Outline For Community Health Work*, Health Education Authority (HEA), 1989
Further Information: Professional and Community Development Division, HEA, Hamilton House, Mabledon Place, London WC1
Telephone 071-383 3833

Main features considered here: Developing a CD curriculum which enables health education workers to incorporate a CD perspective into their work and community development workers to have a health perspective to their work.

Background: As a result of the growing interest over the past few years in a community development approach to health education and promotion local Colleges of Further Education expressed a desire to provide community 'access' courses to their existing Certificate courses in health education. The community health movement was concerned that this would result in a demotion of 'community development' to a minor and lower status aspect of health promotion. The HEA called together a working group on this issue comprising interested people from professional and community settings. As a result a core curriculum for a community health work course emerged, on a full-time or modular basis, along with plans for a conference to place this on the agendas of health education officers, community workers and colleges.

Involvement: The working group has comprised the HEA, the National Community Health Resource (NCHR), the Federation of Community Work Training Groups (FCWTG) and interested community health workers and trainers.

Examples: The course outline for community health work was built on the training needs analysis carried out by the NCHR, the core competences in community work training carried out by the FCWIG and other relevant material based on intensive consultation with community health workers.

Lessons: The working group developing the CD curriculum felt that it was very important that any course was properly accredited by the HEA nationally, to maintain the status of CD.

Title of Project/Work: **Community Involvement in Medical Education at St. Mary's Hospital**

Source of Material: Wendy Farrent *Community Involvement in Medical Education*, Community Health Action, 1988, and *Health For All in the Inner City*, Health Education Authority, 1987

Further Information: Department of Community Medicine, St. Mary's Hospital Medical School, Praed Street, London W2

Main features considered here: Exploring the implications of the principles of community development to undergraduate medical training, with the collaboration of community and voluntary organisations in planning and supervising projects. This was through medical students attending a course in groups during their third or fourth year of medical education. An important part of the course was two weeks' work on a locally based project on an aspect of health promotion policy.

Background: The St. Mary's Lectureship in Health Education was set up through the then Health Education Council to investigate the implications of inner city deprivation for health promotion and community development, especially for medical education.

Involvement: Members of community and voluntary organisations have been centrally involved in designing projects, introducing students to the issues, putting them in touch with relevant agencies and interpreting project findings to be put into action.

Examples: Projects on the district food policy have included working with local Afro-Caribbean organisations in documenting the neglect of food needs of black and ethnic minority groups and collecting information on healthy Afro-Caribbean meals.

Lessons: Students have experienced a more participatory style of research, listening to and learning from local people, gaining insight into the role and workings of the voluntary sector and a wider concept of health promotion.

Title of Project/Work: **Bradford Community Health Forum**
Source of Material: Information from the Health Education Authority

Further Information: Bradford Community Health Forum, c/o 19–25 Sunbridge Road, Bradford BD1 2AY
Telephone 0274 722772

Main features considered here: The Forum has brought together voluntary sector groups and workers with statutory workers such as health visitors and health education officers, who have an interest or involvement in community health issues. It provides information and contact exchange between the different groups, opportunities to share expertise, a newsletter and mailing list and has gained more resources for community health work.
Background: Bradford already had a Community Health Project, but this was based on one estate, while the interest in community health work was citywide. The Community Health Project was increasingly asked to do citywide work eg. providing training and advice. It was felt that providing a Bradford-wide forum would be a more appropriate response.
Involvement: Groups and individuals with an interest in community health work are all involved in the Forum. They have been contacted through word of mouth and via networks such as those of the Council of Voluntary Service and the Community Health Council.
Examples: The Forum has now received funding from the Health Education Authority to link their work to other forums and cities in the Region. Also, when Bradford City Council was considering setting up as a 'Healthy City', the Forum was able to provide ready-made links for a multi-agency strategy.
Lessons: It has been important that all members of the Forum work towards common goals. The existence of the Forum has meant that District and citywide health issues can be dealt with in a way that would not otherwise be possible.

Title of Project/Work: **Cambridge Community Development Health Project (CCDHP)**
Source of Material: CCDHP *A Review of Achievement So Far* and *Community Health Fayres: Recipes for Success* 1989
Further Information: CCDHP, East Barnwell Health Centre, Ditton Lane, Cambridge
Telephone 0223 216666

Main features considered here: Patient participation in the health centre. The CCDHP has two bases, one in a health centre attached to a GP practice, the other in a local neighbourhood. The Practice Participation Association (PPA) was already set up and had initiated a number of self-help groups and a volunteer visiting scheme for the elderly. The Project has worked with the PPA as a major network and a number of new developments have been initiated.
Background: The health centre base was identified for the Project because

of the innovative work done to establish the PPA. Also the City Council had identified the area as being a priority neighbourhood in terms of disadvantage. The Project itself was conceived by the Health Promotion Department of the Health Authority and the City Council Community Services Department to explore community development approaches to health promotion.

Involvement: Original PPA members were identified by GPs and other staff at the health centre. Community involvement is now quite well established and wide ranging.

Examples: The Barnwell Community Health Fayre was conceived by the PPA and organised to meet the aim of participation, furthering community development, involvement, having fun and raising profiles. Other activities include the Community Car Scheme, Women and Depression Group, Women's Health Group and the Swimming Action Group (for the disabled and elderly).

Lessons: There are issues around the PPA and the Project being based at the same centre eg. the physical boundaries of the practice community are not the same as the local neighbourhood community. Conventional methods of evaluation using the medical model are not felt to be useful and so more creative methods are being used eg. making a tape/slide programme.

Title of Project/Work: **'Time for Health' Conference 1989**
Source of Material: Conference material produced by the National Community Health Resource (NCHR)
Further Information: NCHR, 15 Britannia Street, London WC1X 9JP Telephone 071-837 2426

Main features considered here: Organisation of this national four-day conference in Newcastle on 'Community Participation In Health For All By The Year 2000' to consider current health issues in the context of community involvement in health promotion, the reduction of inequalities and ways of professional and community sectors working together. The conference was organised by a combination of national and local professional and community bodies ie. NCHR, Newcastle Community Health Workers, Faculty of Community Medicine, Health Education Authority (HEA), Local Authority Health Network, Association of Community Health Councils and Health Rights.

Background: The organisations involved were invited by the HEA and NCHR to plan an event which would take forward discussion on 'Health For All' between the community health movement and the planners and policy makers. Every aspect of the conference was aimed at putting into practice the three aims of 'Health For All' described above.

Involvement: Besides the range of organisers, around 300 individuals interested in community health from local authorities, health authorities,

large and small voluntary organisations and community groups, attended and participated in the conference.
Examples: The conference was based on a large number of themes or issues. Within each theme, participants met four times with the same group, co-ordinated by two facilitators trained specifically for this purpose. They considered the theme in the context of 'Health For All', sharing skills, knowledge and experience to build their own action plans to take away and to make recommendations about what others could do. Fun events were also planned.
Lessons: A high level of organisational skills was necessary to make the event successful.

Title of Project/Work: **Sheffield Occupational Health Project**
Source of Material: Information from Project Worker
Further Information: Sheffield Occupational Health Project, Birley Moor Health Centre, 1 Eastglade Crescent, Sheffield 12
Telephone 0742 645 691

Main features considered here: The Project works in seven professional practices in Sheffield at primary care level, providing advice to patients on occupational diseases and hazards. Patients are encouraged to improve conditions at work by discussing health and safety problems with other workers and to use straightforward information to raise the level of awareness of hazards. Injured workers or former workers are advised of their compensation rights and of relevant support groups.
Background: There was a growing realisation that many people at work have no access to advice on health and safety. Because primary health care centres are where people go when they are ill, they were seen as the obvious places to discuss the underlying causes of illnesses.
Involvement: The Project seeks to involve workers and community groups in support groups and campaigns around health and safety issues.
Examples: Steelworkers and engineering workers are now improving control of dust and fumes at work partly as a result of the support the Project has given them. Noise control is now a major issue because of the expense to employers' insurers of the Project's campaigns for deafness compensation amongst Yemeni and Bengali workers, miners and others.
Lessons: The Project has shown that disease can be prevented through sufferers or those at risk being given adequate support. Collective methods of tackling health problems work best, in the Project's view, so working with trade unions is effective. It is significant that the Project's workers have experience as shop floor workers themselves and/or appropriate scientific or technical training.

Strategic support
Title of Project/Work: **Professional and Community Development (PCD) Division of the Health Education Authority (HEA)**
Source of Material: HEA PCD Division *Operational Plan 1988/89*; HEA *Ministerial Review of Community Development 1989*
Further Information: PCD Division, HEA, Hamilton House, Mabledon Place, London WC1
Telephone 071-383 3833

Main features considered here: Policy development by a Division within a national statutory health agency to strategically develop and promote Community Development in health. In practice this includes building a broadly-based infrastructure, encouraging the opening up of policy making procedures, promoting principles and actions and developing knowledge of Community Development in health.
Background: In 1988 the HEA, as a new statutory Health Authority, established a new Division to promote professional and community development in health education nationally.
Involvement: The PCD Division works through national and local statutory and voluntary agencies, health professionals and community health workers.
Examples: The Division have advised the Oxford Regional Health Authority on its CD strategy for health promotion by helping devise a project for the Region, advising on appropriate pilot projects and helping monitor, evaluate and disseminate the results.
Lessons: The Division has had to work on at least two levels simultaneously, always drawing in and co-operating with others, to make progress; the public relations level of making large institutions receptive to new approaches in health promotion, and the professional/community level of building up an infrastructure so this receptiveness can be taken advantage of.

Title of Project/Work: **National Self-help Support Centre (NSHSC)**
Source of Material: NSHSC *A Report of the First Two Years 1988;* NSHSC *Bulletin Mutual Aid and Self-Help* 1986
Further Information: NSHSC, National Council for Voluntary Organisations, 26 Bedford Square, London WC1B 3HU
Telephone 071-636 4066

Main features considered here: Provision of strategic support to self-help groups by fostering support and focusing national attention on the need for such support. This takes place through its information service, development of networks, training programme, contact with professionals and publications.
Background: The NSHSC was established in 1986 in response to an

upsurge of interest in self-help groups in the fields of health and social services.
Involvement: Members include national and local workers supporting self-help groups, policy makers, researchers and others concerned to develop support for self-help groups.
Examples: The NSHSV has established networks to overcome isolation, share common worries and for mutual learning. One of these is the Black and Ethnic Minority Self-Help Workers Network, networking round issues such as funding, survival strategies within white organisations, not allowing divisions among communities, manipulating power structures, and not becoming 'buffers' between institutions and self-help groups. Other networks are the National Self-Help Support Network for local workers and the network for representatives of national specialist self-help organisations.
Lessons: The NSHSC is planning to continue the above and share experience with self-help support initiatives in fields such as education, arts, unemployment and neighbourhood action.

Title of Project/Work: **Leeds City Council Health Unit**
Source of Material: Information from Project Worker
Further Information: Leeds City Council Health Unit, 2nd Floor Annexe, Civil Hall, Leeds LS1 3AQ
Telephone 0532 462431

Main features considered here: The Unit provides support by bringing together statutory agencies in a working party to draw up a joint health promotion strategy for Leeds which will take it towards 'Health For All' by the year 2000 and by financing two pilot Community Development projects. The working party and the projects feed directly into the Joint Consultative Committee (JCC) and its strategy work. This has resulted in the Leeds Action Plan which has eleven recommendations as a starting point, including appointing local Development Officers from within communities, drawing up a health profile, developing training materials to initiate and support public participation and allocating ten per cent of joint finance for developing public participation initiatives which promote inter-sectoral collaboration.
Background: The Health Unit was set up in 1986 as a response to the City Council's desire to put health higher on their agenda and to the extreme under-resourcing of the Health Education service in the area. The Unit soon decided to draw in as many agencies as possible through the JCC (joint between the Local and Health Authority) to look at a joint strategy for Leeds.
Involvement: Representatives from community and voluntary organisations are represented on the sub groups of the JCC which fed into the Action

Plan. The recommendations are designed to promote the involvement of the community in setting the agendas and targets via the local development projects.

Examples: The Unit set up an advocacy service which tries to give a more equal voice to disadvantaged people in the city by helping them to gain access to services and to put their needs forward.

Lessons: It takes a long time to genuinely involve lots of people, because of the importance of getting professionals to a common starting point for health promotion while allowing community people to set the agenda. Inter-sectoral training can help this process.

Title of Project/Work: **Yorkshire Regional Health Authority (RHA) Health Promotion Office**
Source of Material: RHA Health Promotion, *Guidelines For Districts On Community Health Promotion*
Further Information: Health Promotion Office, Yorkshire RHA, Park Parade, Harrogate HG1 5AH
Telephone 0423 500066

Main features considered here: Providing strategic support for community health promotion at Regional level through the Community Health Promotion Sub Group of the Regional Health Promotion Group, which was set up on a multi-disciplinary basis. This sub group surveyed a sample number of District Health Authorities on the support they give community health initiatives. They also surveyed Community Health Councils on their views of health promotion work. From their findings, they drew up a set of guidelines for Districts on community health promotion. This was also informed by material from the national conference on community health education for health education officers in Bradford.

Background: Community health promotion was one of the priority areas originally put forward by the Regional Health Promotion Group.

Involvement: The sub group comprises representatives from the Regional Association of Community Health Councils, as well as health professionals working in the community, such as health education officers, GPs and health visitors. There are no direct representatives from community groups, although this is suggested for local forums.

Examples: The *Guidelines* have twelve recommendations for Districts, one of which is about evaluation. This makes the point that evalution needs to be qualitative, participatory, reflecting processes and goals and should have a long timescale to allow for flexibility and change.

Lessons: The group feels that further support may be necessary for Districts to pursue the *Guidelines* and there will need to be discussions with the Health Education Authority.

Title of Project/Work: **Consortium on Opportunities for Volunteering**
Source of Material: Information from Project Worker
Further Information: Consortium on Opportunities For Volunteering, c/o 26 Bedford Square, London WC1
Telephone 071-580 6387

Main features considered here: Co-ordinating the General Fund of money from the Department of Health and Social Security (DHSS) to support local projects in the health and social welfare field, as one of sixteen National Agencies. The Consortium has responsibility for administering the Fund and allocating grants to projects which involve unemployed volunteers in their work.
Background: The 'Opportunities For Volunteering' Scheme was set up by the DHSS in 1982 as a 'one-year, one-off' central government initiative. Ten national voluntary networks came together to form the Consortium to administer the Fund. It is now a three-year rolling programme with £5½ million per year available for funding local projects.
Involvement: The local projects which receive funding are run by voluntary management committees drawn from and involving volunteers from the local community. The projects themselves are responsible for electing management committees and recruiting and selecting volunteers.
Examples: In awarding grants the Consortium favours groups working towards a deliberate policy of equal opportunities. Current priorities include projects involving black and ethnic minority communities, women and people with disabilities, and projects which meet the needs of those living in rural areas.
Lessons: It has been important in allocating grants to projects, to provide money for volunteers' out of pocket expenses, staff costs and office expenses, training, project equipment, vehicles and minor renovation work to ensure access for disabled people.

Title of Project/Work: **Federation of Community Work Training Groups (FCWTG)**
Source of Material: FCWTG *Annual Report 1989*
Further Information: FCWTG, 356 Glossop Road, Sheffield S10 2HW
Telephone 0742 739391

Main features considered here: Promoting community development through the identification of basic skills and applying these to training. This work was undertaken with the support of fourteen Regional Community Work Training Groups and as part of the development of community work training nationally.
Background: The Federation has been operating for eight years through a regional structure to ensure that community development plays a consistent part in the lives of individuals, groups and communities. This grew out of

its work on the accreditation of learning through experience of community work. Recently it has assisted in the development of a community health work course for the Health Education Authority.

Involvement: The Federation combines fourteen regional training groups, each of which consists of a range of people doing community work on a paid or voluntary basis, on a range of issues including health, and who are interested in promoting and developing community work training.

Examples: 1988/89 has been a significant year for the accreditation work as two accreditation units, Greater Manchester and West of Scotland, have published the outcomes of their pilot accreditation programmes. Fourteen people have now had their experience accredited by the FCWTG. Also this work has been linked with establishing basic skills for community work.

Lessons: It has been vital that the FCWTG's work on skills has in turn been based on the experience of existing community workers, groups and organisations and that it has been able to relate these different fields involved with community development. Co-operation with the HEA has been important in promoting community development training in health.

Title of Project/Work: **Oxford Regional Health Authority (RHA) Health Promotion Department**
Source of Material: Information from Oxford RHA
Further Information: Oxford RHA Health Promotion Department, Old Road, Headington, Oxford OX3 7LF
Telephone 0865 64861

Main features considered here: Funding community-based health projects for a minimum of two years covering very small and defined geographical areas within three District Health Authorities and managed by those Districts. The areas are selected according to criteria of relative deprivation. The primary aim is to seek community views on factors influencing their health and to achieve change in those areas through applying resources intensively, thereby improving health. The intersectoral nature of the projects is stressed.

Background: In 1985/86 the RHA carried out a life survey in several Districts. The data revealed that there were certain areas deprived socially in health terms. It was felt that traditional health education methods would not be successful in improving health status equally across social classes and in fact may help to exacerbate class differences. As a response the Region put aside around £200,000 from its Health Promotion Fund to fund three community-based health projects within the three most deprived areas.

Involvement: Each project now employs community health workers or coordinators with the key task of involving residents, through working with community groups, leafletting, public meetings and existing networks of health and social welfare workers. In Northampton, for instance, the

community are involved with policy and planning as well as implementation.
Examples: In Milton Keynes the involvement of other agencies in the work has been so impressive that the Development Corporation have agreed to fund the evaluation.
Lessons: There was a need from the outset to be as definitive as possible about aims, methods, tasks and evalution in order to justify clearly the intentions and effects of the work.

Title of Project/Work: **King's Fund Carers' Unit**
Source of Material: King's Fund Carers Unit *The Informal Caring Support Programme - A Briefing Paper* and *A New Deal For Carers* 1989
Further Information: Carers' Unit, King's Fund Centre, 126 Albert Street, London NW1 7NF
Telephone 071-267 6111

Main features considered here: Supporting informal carers nationally through consulting carers and their organisations about priority needs, developing and disseminating information, working with Health and Local Authorities and voluntary organisations to encourage better support services and reinforcing and developing networks of individuals and organisations concerned with carers.
Background: Throughout the 1980s, awareness of the significance of carers and the disadvantages for them in current community care arrangements grew. Government recognition of this led to the funding and establishment of the Carers' Unit in 1986.
Involvement: People became involved in the Unit's advisory groups through open invitations to help develop the work. They are individual carers, voluntary organisations and community groups concerned with carers including those from black and ethnic minority groups, and a wide range of community workers and front line staff in health and social services.
Examples: The development of 'A New Deal For Carers' came about through the National Caring Forum, a group of voluntary organisations convened by the Unit to feed in carers' views. The Forum met regularly with the Unit to proactively put forward suggestions and ideas and to disseminate the resulting work to a wide range of carers.
Lessons: Building up trust, confidence and joint working possibilities with voluntary organisations and community groups has been crucial in identifying community needs and enabling interested individuals to participate in the Unit's work at national and local level. It is this which has enabled the Unit to reach out to the large dispersed carer population.

Section 3: Structured Bibliography

Community Development for Health: The British Experience

Section A. Reports on Individual Local CDH Projects

A major feature of the literature on community development for health in Britain is the wealth of reports on individual projects, often reports that have been produced internally, but that have had a much wider circulation and readership on informal networks.

1 *The Albany Health Project, Deptford, East London*
This was one of the earliest initiatives in Britain, starting in 1977, and based in the Albany Community and Social Action Centre, in an area of long-standing urban decay. The first stages were reported on in:
Kathy Tetlow, Deptford's Community Health Project, *Medicine in Society*, 1979, Vol. 5, No. 4, pp. 16–21.
A series of annual reports provide interesting details of the Project's work and a useful retrospective is found in:
The Albany Health Project, *The First Five Years*, The Albany, Douglas Way, Deptford London SE8, 24pp/A4.

2 *The Bethnal Green Health Project, East London*
This began in 1982, with a basis in one of the longest-established community settlements in London, Oxford House (which dates back to 1884).
A leaflet, an information sheet, and a report on the first three years' work are available from the Project, at Oxford House, Derbyshire Street, Bethnal Green, London E2 6HG.

3 *Catford Community Health Project, East London*
This was initiated by the Community Health Council in Lewisham, and was closely associated with an experimental neighbourhood scheme called Catford Link. It began in 1982, and a detailed evaluation report was published in 1985:
Liz Reason, *Catford Community Health Project Evaluation Report*, December 1985, Catford CHP, 17pp/A4.

4 *Glasgow*
Two initiatives are notable here. One is based in a NHS setting:
Sue Laughlin & David Black, *Improving Health in areas of Disadvantage-Community Strategy of the Health Education Department*, Greater Glasgow Health Board, Health Education Department, May 1986, 12pp/A4.

The other is the Glasgow Community Health Resource, supported by the Strathclyde Regional Council.
They have produced a Review of their first two years' work (1988) and they publish a newsletter, of which Issue No. 3 (March 1989) focuses on community participation in healthy cities.

5 *Glyndon Health Project, Greenwich, East London*
This was started in 1985 by Greenwich Community Health Council, as part of a broader 'Health Rights Project', to enable people in the Glyndon ward to get more information about their own health and to improve local services. A brief article appeared as:
Graeme Betts & Deborah Loeb, The Glyndon Health Project, *Radical Community Medicine 1987*, Spring No. 29, pp. 52-4.
A fuller report is available:
Glyndon Health Project, *Annual Report 1987-88*, Greenwich CHC 23, Anglesea Road, London SE18 6EG, 29pp/A4.

6 *Homerton Community Health Project, Hackney, East London*
This began in 1981, in a highly deprived area of North-East London, on the initiative of the City and Hackney Community Health Council with funds from the Inner City Partnership.
Information sheets and leaflets are available, and there is a highly informative 'Activities Report' covering the period 1981–1983, called *Health in Homerton*, 40pp/A4.

7 *Mansfield Community Health Project*
This project is located in a small market town in the mining area of the East Midlands. It began in 1982, within a general community development project established by Nottinghamshire Social Services and the (national) Community Projects Foundation. From 1982 there was funding from the Health Education Council. Two reports are available:
Mansfield Community Health Project, Nottinghamshire County Council with the Health Education Council, May 1984, 20pp/A4.
The Ripples, a report of a joint funded project between the Health Education Council and Nottinghamshire County Council Social Services Department, 1986, 105pp/A4.

8 *Myatts Field Health Project, South London*
This Project was based on a large new housing estate in North Brixton in Lambeth, and the worker was located in the newly-opened health centre on the estate. A report on three years work is available:
Theresa Jerome, *Myatts Field Health Project: Project Workers Report*, 1987 (available at NCHR), 22pp/A4.

9 Paddington & North Kensington Health Authority Projects, West London

The Health Education Department in this Authority was the location for a lengthy series of pioneering initiatives in CDH, reported on as follows:

Charles Manicom & John Dodds, *A Community Development Approach within a Health Education Department*, paper for HEC Conference, York, March 1981 16pp/A4.

Public Health Advisory Service, with Alan Beattie, *Paddington Health Audit* Project, Final Report, March, 1982, 34pp/A4.

John Dodds & Jean Spray, *Evolving Practice in Health Education*, paper for Faculty of Community Medicine Conference, Autumn 1984, 16pp/A4.

Vari Drennan, 'A New Approach', *Nursing Mirror* 1984 Oct. 17 Vol. 159, No. 14.

Vari Drennan, *Working in a Different Way: community work methods and health visiting*, PNKHA, May 1985, 86pp/A4.

Vari Drennan, *Effective Health Education in the Inner-City: Report of a Feasibility Study examining Community Development Approaches for Health Education Officers and Health Education Departments*, PNKHA, June 1986, 86pp/A4.

Wendy Farrant, *Health for All in the Inner City: Proposed Framework for a Community Development Approach to Health Promotion Policy and Planning at District Level*, PNKHA, April, 1986, 30pp/A4.

Wendy Farrant & Angela Taft, 'Building Healthy Public Policy in an unhealthy, political climate: a case study from Paddington and North Kensington', *Health Promotion*, 1988, Vol. 3, No. 3, pp. 287–292.

10 The Peckham Health Project, South London

This was a very early initiative which lasted for four years from 1977 to 1981, and was based at a local settlement, located within a community centre. There was an informative interim report in 1979 and the community worker and the general practitioner who were prominent in the project subsequently wrote a useful retrospective review:

Maggie Cochrane & Brian Fisher, 'Peckham Health Project: Raising Health Consciousness', *Community Development Journal*, 1983, Vol. 18, No. 2, April, pp. 177–181.

11 Newcastle Community Health Projects

Newcastle-upon-Tyne in North-East England has been the home of several substantial initiatives. These have been reviewed in a wide-ranging evaluation report:

Christopher Pollitt, *An Evaluation of the Community Health Projects at Walker, North Kenton and Riverside*, October 1984, 68pp/A4.

The individual projects also produce their own annual reports; and the Riverside Project has been the focus of two other special reports:

The Riverside Child Health Project Evaluation Report, 1983, Department of Family & Community Medicine, University of Newcastle upon Tyne, 208pp/A4.

How We Feel about Working with Groups: Report by locally recruited Group Convenors at Riverside Child Health Project, The Project, October 1984, 12pp/A4.

12 Nottingham Health Education Unit

This Unit established community development work as a consistent function within the Unit, with a specialist Health Education Officer post, from 1981 onwards. Relevant reviews include:

Neil Boot, *Promoting Health with Community Groups*, Nottingham Practical Papers in Health Education, No. 10, Nottingham University/Nottingham Health Education Unit, 1984, 26pp/A4.

Neil Boot, 'Community Health Action challenges for the health education officer', *Health Education Journal* 1985, Vol. 44, No. 4, pp. 203–207.

13 Salford Community Health Project

This initiative is set in a Health Authority context, and a detailed report of its first three years is available:

Linda Youd & Liz Jayne, *Salford Community Health Project: the First Three Years*, Salford CHP, 1986, 28pp/A4.

14 Sheffield Community Health Projects

An early initiative in the South Yorkshire city of Sheffield, based in a health centre, was reported on as follows:

Jane Greetham, Community Development through a Community Health Project, Association of Community Workers *Talking Point* No. 40, December 1982, 5pp/A4.

A later project has been joint funded by Sheffield City Council, Sheffield Health Authority, and the Health Education Authority, starting in 1987. The most recent report gives a detailed descriptive account of its activities:

Sharrow Community Health Project, *Second Report*, January 1989, 15pp/A4.

15 The Stockwell Health Project, South London

This inner city area was the location for a project, based within the Lady Margaret Hall Settlement, which produced a series of reports between 1980 and 1984:

Mawbey Brough: a Health Centre for the Community? January 1980; second edition June 1982, 24pp/A4.

Stockwell Health Project: After Two Years, September 1982, 30pp/A4.

Health Matters: A Report on the Work of the Stockwell Health Project 1982-3, 12pp/A4.

Juliet Coke, *A Focus on Health and Race - Mawbey Brough Community Health: a Case Study*, Community Service Volunteers, December 1984, 32pp/A4.

16 *Thornhill Neighbourhood Project, North London*
This initiative, in Islington, was a broad-based community project, in which health became a major focus of activity. Two reports illustrate this:
Health Care in Thornhill: a case of inner city deprivation, May 1978, 15pp/A4.
Antenatal Care - Who Benefits? A Report by Thornhill Neighbourhood Project, June, 1982, 48pp/A4.

17 *Waterloo Health Project, South London*
This was one of the three pioneering initiatives in South London in the late 1970s (along with the Albany and the Peckham projects). It had its origins in a community education centre, but subsequently gained support from the local authority Social Services Department in Lambeth with Inner City Partnership funding. There was a series of informative annual reports; then a retrospective review:
Six Years of Community Health Struggles: Report of the Waterloo Health Project, Waterloo Health Project, 1983, 30pp/A4.

18 *West Lambeth Children's Health Club, South London*
This initiative was located within a Community Health Council setting, focused on 'peer-teaching', and was the subject of a very thorough evaluation, which created widespread interest at the time. See:
Lesley Levane, Alan Beattie, Diane Plamping & Sue Thorne, *St Thomas Children's Health Club: a Report*, King's Fund, 1981, 46pp/A4.
Plamping D, Thorne S & Gelbier S, 'Peer Teaching in Health Education', *British Dental Journal*, 1980, Vol. 149, pp. 113-115.
Smith R, 'Health education by children for children', *British Medical Journal* 1981, Vol. 583 782.
Plamping D, 'Learning from children learning: peer tutoring in health education, *Radical Community Medicine*, 1986, Summer No. 26, pp. 31-40.

19 *Whiteway Health Project, Bath*
This initiative was prompted by a joint planning team between the Health Authority and the Social Services Dept in Bath. It is based on a council housing estate. Two reports describe the work of the Project:
Whiteway Health Project: The First Year, February 1985, 28pp/A4.
Whiteway Health Project Annual Report, 1986.
Vivienna Aird, 'Whiteway Health Project: an example of a community development approach to health care', *Radical Health Promotion*, 1987, 6, pp. 3-6.

20 *Winchester Project*
This was initiated by the National Children's Bureau, focusing on education for parenthood in one neighbourhood – a council housing estate in Winchester. It was fully monitored during its three years of activity 1983–6: Gillian Pugh & Lin Poulton, *Parenting as a Job for Life: a local development project in Hampshire*, National Children's Bureau, January 1987, 100pp/A4.

Section B: Reports on CDH projects with particular interest groups

Several of the local projects listed in Section A have focused at least at some stage on the health circumstances of particular social groups; but there are a few projects which make the health disadvantages of a particular group their principal focus:

B.1 Women's health
One project listed above with a partial focus on women's health is the Thornhill project (16).

21 Caroline Leinster, *What We Need Is Women, Health and the Health Service in Newcastle in Tyne*, the Primary Health Care Project, 1981–83, Newcastle Inner City Forum and Newcastle Community Health Council, July 1983, 120pp/A4.
Reports an investigation of the views of six different women's groups concerning services for mothers and toddlers in the community.

22 Sue Dowling, *Health for a Change: the provision of preventative health care in pregnancy and early childhood*, Child Poverty Action Group, 1983, 74pp/A5.
This brings together case studies of new ways of reaching parents of under-fives, and highlights the benefits of voluntary action and community participation.

23 Rosemary Allen & Andrew Purkis, *Health in the Round: Voluntary Action and antenatal services*, NCVO, 1983, 104pp/A4.
Provides a map of what voluntary organisations and volunteers are doing for parents-to-be up and down the country, argues for bolder investment in voluntary action, including parent participation and describes several successful initiatives.

24 Workers Education Association, *Women's Health Resource Pack*, WEA/HEA, 1988.
Brings together a range of ideas and resources for working with women in a participative way on health issues, drawing on experience in a Manchester WEA project.

B.2 Health of black & ethnic minority groups

One project listed above with a partial focus on black and ethnic minority health is that at Mawbey Brough, Stockwell (15).

25 Asma Ahmad, Maggie Pearson & Ruth Evans, *Multi-racial initiatives in Maternity Care*, Maternity Alliance, 1985, 112pp/A4.
Reports a survey of thirty four initiatives – the majority undertaken by voluntary groups – which seek to improve the accessibility and quality of parental and child health services to black and ethnic minority users. The importance of collaboration between statutory services and the community is underlined.

26 Jocelyn Cornwell & Pat Gordon, *Experiment in Advocacy: The Hackney Multi-ethnic Womens Health Project*, King's Fund Paper, 84/237, 1984.
Describes a project which weas based in a CHC, and was prompted by concerns about antenatal care for non-English-speaking women. It developed a scheme of local 'patient advocates', emphasising cooperation between the health service and the community.

27 Allan McNaught, *Health Action and Ethnic Minorities*, National Community Health Resource (NCHR), 1987, 74pp/A5.
A review commissioned by NCHR, of the contribution of community initiatives to the development of local health services that are more responsive to the needs of ethnic minority people. Outlines a strategy for establishing and supporting such initiatives.

28 Usha Prashar, Elizabeth Anionwu, Micha Brozovic, *Sickle Cell Anaemia: Who Cares?* Runnymede Trust, 1985.
Reports a survey of services for sickle cell disease in English health authorities and draws attention to the vital role of local centres with voluntary/community support.

29 World Health Organisation, Community Control of Hereditary Anaemias, *Bullet. WHO*, 1983, 63(1), pp. 63–80.
A memo from the WHO meeting which recommends cooperation between voluntary groups and statutory services in connection with the sickle cell and thalessemia syndromes, citing successful initiatives in Britain and other European countries.

B.3 Health of older people

30 Jan Smith, *Positive Health Skills for Older People: a Community-based Approach*, Report of First Stage, July 1985; Report of the Second and

Third Stages, December 1985, Bradford and Airedale Health Education Unit, Shipley, West Yorkshire, 40pp/A4.
Offers a profile of 100 community-based groups of older people. Explains how they operate, and suggests ways in which resources and networks can be built up.

31 Maggie Jee, *Health in Retirement (Fulham North): Interim Evaluation of a Community Development Project for Older People*, Bishop Creighton House Settlement, London, April 1988, 23pp/A4.
An interim report (after two years' work) on a CD project aimed at supporting health promotion schemes and health-related activities with older people in West London.

32 Health Education Authority, *Age Well Ideas Pack*, HEA/NCHR, 2nd edition, 1989.
A set of worksheets drawing on the successful experience of community-based health projects with older people throughout Britain.

B.4 Health of young people

Three local projects listed above which have a focus on children's health are those at Riverside, Newcastle (11); West Lambeth (18); and Winchester (20).

33 Robyn Gorna, *Community-based AIDS Initiatives in the UK*, Community Projects Foundation/Health Education Authority, 1989.
A review of how the community approach has so far been applied in HIV/AIDS work in the UK.

34 Fiona Reynoldson, *Grapevine: a Review of the FPA's North London-based community project for young people 1971–1981*, Family Planning Association, Project Report No. 2, 1982.
Summarizes the first ten years of a pioneering project which developed the peer teaching principle in sex education work with young people.

35 *Ideals and Realities: a consumers' evaluation of a community mental health project:* Forty-Second Street, Youth Development Trust, Manchester, 1984, 24pp/A4.
Presents a profile of the users' reactions to a local project for young people under stress.

Section C: Reports on CDH in particular professional contexts

Some of the literature on CDH that has already been cited refers to studies of this approach to health promotion within the work of particular professional groups. See for example under reference 9 above, Manicom and Dodds, and Dodds and Spray (who report on CDH in the work of Health Education Officers), and Drennan (who reports on CDH in the work of Health Visitors and of Health Education Officers). Also, under reference 12, see Boot on CDH in a Health Education Unit. Additional publications are as follows:

36 Diana Balter, Hasel Daniels, Jenny Finch & Elizabeth Perkins, *Training Health Visitors in Work with Community Groups*, Nottingham Practical Papers in Health Education No. 14, University of Nottingham/Nottingham Health Education Unit, 1986, 40pp/A4.
Gives an account of the development and evaluation of an experimental course for health visitors on working with community groups.

37 Alison Watt, Community Health Initiatives and their relationship to general practice, *Journal of the Royal College of General Practitioners*, 1986 (February) No. 36, pp. 72–73.
Reviews the community health movement and suggests six ways in which GPs can help and support local voluntary action on health.

38 Wendy Farrant, *Health for All in the Inner City: exploring the implications for medical education*, Paper for Health Education Council Workshop on Health Promotion in the Medical Undergraduate Curriculum, Sheffield University, March 1987, 10pp/A4.
Describes a range of projects undertaken at St Mary's Hospital Medical School in which undergraduate medical students were given experience of community participation on health issues in an inner-city area.

Section D: Directories and compilations of CDH projects

Publications of this sort have been a prominent and useful resource for those working in the CDH field in recent years. The earlier examples are mainly of historical interest by now, and a chronological listing seems appropriate.

39 Caroline Smith, *Community Based Health Initiatives: a handbook for voluntary groups*, National Council for Voluntary Organizations (NCVO) 1982, 34pp/A4.
Reviews 'current practice' by summarizing nine projects around Britain, and identifying useful 'starting points' for new groups.

40 Caroline Smith, *Directory of Community Health Initiatives*, NCVO 1st edition January 1982; 2nd edition November 1982, 33pp/A4.
Brings together self-descriptions of local projects in Britain (outside Greater London) – more than forty in the 1st edition, more than sixty in the 2nd.

41 Jean Spray, Helen Rosenthal & Mai Wann, *Community Initiatives in Health Education*, London Community Health Resource, June 1983, 31pp/A4.
Reports a survey of seventeen projects (sixteen in London) to illustrate the variety of activity taking place at local level in different areas.

42 Julia Chaplin & Durrah Adams, *London Health Action Network*, 4th edition, 1986, 49pp/A4.
Complements reference 40 above, by providing information on community health initiatives in the Greater London area – over 150 of them.

43 Charmian Kenner, *Whose Needs Count? Community Action for Health*, NCVO, 1986, 110pp/A5.
A survey commissioned by CHIRU of ten selected community health initiatives in England, drawing on interviews with project workers and users, and indicating points of overlap with self-help projects.

44 Community Health Initiatives Resource Unit/London Community Health Resource *Guide to Community Health Projects* CHIRU/LCHR, 1987, 128pp/A4.
Reviews definitions of community health projects, reports a national survey of thirty three projects, and offers guidelines for setting up projects.

45 Lesley Saunders (Ed), *Action for Health: Initiatives in Local Communities*, Community Projects Foundation/Health Education Authority/Scottish Health Education Group, 1988, 209pp/A5.
Drawing on the experience of twenty five projects, examines the history of their growth, the forms they take, and the issues they tackle.

Section E: Theoretical commentaries on CDH

Any sort of consistent or coherent framework for discussion and decision-making about CDH has been slow in coming in Britain, in spite of the wealth of practical experience arising from local projects. The contributions listed below are therefore heterogeneous and differ considerably in the depth and rigour with which they examine conceptual issues:

46 Lee Adams, 'Community Development and Health Education', *Radical Health Promotion* No. 3, Winter 1986, pp. 23–26.
Sets out a map of the advantages and disadvantages of the CDH approach for health workers.

47 Alan Beattie, 'Community Development for Health: from Practice to Theory?' *Radical Health Promotion* No. 4, Summer 1986, pp. 12–18.
Suggests there are four distinct alternative models in operation within CDH

work – community outreach, community empowerment, community coordination, and community action – and argues that different relations of power and control are embedded in these models.

48 David Black, 'Community Development and Health Issues', *Radical Health Promotion* No. 1, Spring 1985, pp. 16–19.
Examines the rationale for CDH as an essential direction for health education in areas of multiple deprivation, written from the standpoint of a health education officer (in Glasgow).

49 Lynette Domoney, Gerry Smale & John Warwick, *Community Social Work and Health Promotion*, National Institute for Social Work, 1989, 14pp/A4.
Report of a feasibility study carried out for the Health Education Authority which set out to map areas where partnership between social services and health services is crucial to health promotion and community development.

50 Wendy Farrant, 'Health for WHO by the Year 2000? Choices for district health promotion strategies', *Radical Community Medicine*, 1986/7, Winter, pp. 19–26.
Suggests that while 'Health for All' can legitimise a participatory approach to health promotion, the medical paradigm persists in seizing the health targets and ignoring community participation as a way of working.

51 Stephen Hatch & Ilona Kickbusch, *Self-help and Health in Europe*, WHO, 1984.
Brings together twenty four case studies from twelve countries (including Britain) on self-help initiatives in relation to statutory health services. It offers pointers to the similarities and differences between self-help and community development for health.

52 Eileen Hornsey, 'Informal Approaches to Health Education', *Outlines*, Community Education Development Centre, 1981, 3pp/A4.
A brief note which links CDH projects to the 'informal' approaches familiar in the adult and community education field.

53 John Hubley, 'Community Education, Community Development and Health Education', *Community Education*, 1978/9, Winter, pp. 129–33.
John Hubley, *A Community Development Approach to Health Education in a Multiply-deprived Community in Scotland*, Paper for 10th International Conference on Health Education, London, September 1979, 15pp/A4.
John Hubley, *Community Health Projects in London: Report on a Study Tour*, Paisley College, Scotland, July 1980, 20pp/A4.

John Hubley, 'Community Development and Health Education', *Journal of the Institute of Health Education*, 1980, No. 18, 8pp.
John Hubley, *Health, Informal Education, and the Community Outlines*, Community Education Development Centre, 1981, 3pp/A4.
A series of papers by one of the earliest advocates of CDH in Britain: connections are made to wider debates on generic community work; on the sociology of public health; and on adult/informal education.

54 Jane Jones, *Community Development and Health Issues: a review of existing theory and practice*, Community Projects Foundation, Edinburgh, January 1983, 50pp/A4.
Jane Jones, 'Community Development and Health Promotion: who is WHO talking to? *Radical Community Medicine*, 1987, Summer, pp. 35–38.
Written by an experienced community health worker from Edinburgh. The first paper reports on a three-month study of eighteen projects in England and Scotland, which are discussed in relation to wider issues in public health, medical sociology, and health education. The second paper argues that CDH projects are vital in creating a climate for participation but are struggling against enormous odds.

55 Angela Kilian, 'Conscientisation: an empowering, non-formal education approach for community health workers', *Community Development Journal*, 1988, Vol. 23, No. 2, pp. 117–123.
Draws parallels between CDH and the ideas of Freire and other adult education theorists, and explores these concepts in interviews with community health workers on six projects in London.

56 Jill Rakusen, 'Community Health Projects', *Voluntary Action*, 1982, Winter, pp. 24–25.
A brief review of community health projects in Britain – definitions, aims, difficulties, and achievements.

57 Helen Rosenthal, *Health and Community Work – some new approaches*, King's Fund Report KF 80/117, May 1980, 15pp/A4.
Helen Rosenthal, 'Neighbourhood Health Projects – some new approaches to health and community work in parts of the United Kingdom', *Community Development Journal*, 1983, Vol. 18, No. 2, April, pp. 120–131.
Highly influential papers by someone who helped to initiate local projects and subsequently to establish the London Community Health Resource (in 1981). The papers review eight pioneering projects and relate them to wider literature on community work and on the politics of health.

58 Alex Scott-Samuel, 'Community Development, "Outreach" and Health Association of Community Workers' *Talking Point* No. 33, March 1982, 6pp.
An early review of projects in England by a specialist in community medicine who has supported the community health movement: identifies appropriate issues for local action and discusses collaboration with medical experts.

59 Kasturi Sen, *Training for Health Education through Community Development*, London Community Health Resource, July 1985, 38pp/A4.
A report on a study commissioned by the Health Education Council, carried out at LCHR, to assess the training needs of workers within community health projects, and to determine appropriate ways of providing training.

60 Margaret Stacey, 'Strengthening Communities', *Health Promotion*, 1987, Vol. 2, No. 4, pp. 317–321.
Written by an eminent pioneer of the sociology of 'community', it examines and approves some of the recent work in CDH in Britain.

61 Pat Thornley, 'Community Participation – Rhetoric or Reality?' *Community Health Action*, 1988, Summer, Issue 9, pp. 7–10.
Written from the experience of a community-based women's health project in Liverpool, this paper is critical of the rhetoric of community particiption within the 'Healthy Cities' initiative; it suggests that CDH is in danger of elitist takeover and institutionalisation.

62 Alison Watt, *Community Health Initiatives: clarifying the complexities within the community health movement*, paper for King's Fund Conference 'Community Development in Health', KF/LCHR/CHIRU, January, 1986.
Alison Watt, 'Community Health Education: a time for caution?' Chapter 8 in Sue Rodmell & Alison Watt (eds.), *The Politics of Health Education*, Routledge 1986.
Alison Watt, 'Room for Movement? The Community Response to Medical Dominance', *Radical Community Medicine*, 1987, Spring, pp. 40–45.
Alison Watt & Sue Rodmell, 'Community Involvement in Health Promotion: Progress or Panacea?' *Health Promotion*, 1988, Vol. 2, No. 4, pp. 359–367.
Written from experience as a community health worker and health education officer, these papers express reservations about the vagaries of the community health movement at several levels: confusion over aims and strategies; over-generalised use of the word 'community'; and professional takeover of CDH as a rhetoric by expert groups, to the exclusion of lay people.

63 Yorkshire Regional Health Authority Health Promotion, *Community Health Education: A Time To Take Stock* NCHR 1987, 80pp/A4.
This is a full report of the proceedings of the first National Community Health Action Conference, held in Bradford in April 1986; summarises main sessions and more than fifty workshops, illustrating a wide range of debate and innovation.

Section F: Evaluation of CDH projects

Issues of strategy and methodology in evaluating success and failures in CDH projects have loomed large in many of the individual project reports cited above. Notable examples of ingenious investigation and/or reportage are Albany (1), Catford (3), Mansfield (7), Drennan in 1985 and 1986 at Paddington (9), Pollitt and the Riverside study in Newcastle (11), Salford (13), Sharrow in Sheffield (14), Coke at Stockwell (15), Waterloo (17), West Lambeth (18), Whiteways in Bath (19), Winchester (20), Jee in Fulham (31), Manchester (35). There are also a few publications which review evaluation issues in CDH work, in relation to wider debates in the evaluation of health services, community education, etc.

64 Alan Beattie, 'Evaluating Community Health Initiatives', an Overview Paper for the Conference *Community Development in Health: addressing the confusions*, King's Fund/CHIRU/LCHR, 1984, pp. 23-37.
An extensive review, drawing on current examples of evaluation in CDH, and drawing parallels with wider fields of evaluation work; suggests that there are four different strategies – measuring outcomes; monitoring processes; analysing client perspectives; and appraising institutional agendas – and argues that evaluation needs to become more multi-faceted.
Alan Beattie, 'From Quantity to Quality? The 4E's of evaluation', *Community Health Action* 1989, 12 (Spring), pp. 1-9.
Relates attempts to evaluate CDH projects to recent debates on 'Performance Review' in the statutory sector; and suggests that in CDH the mixed bag of evaluation must include attention to the questions of social ethics that are central to local health action.

65 Lois Graessle & Su Kingsley, *Measuring change, Making changes: an approach to evaluation*, LCHR 1986, 25pp/A4.
A report which arose out of a course on evaluation for community health workers, organised by LCHR. It covers: What is evaluation? Who is it for and what do they want? When do you do it? Who does it? Why bother? It also suggests stages for the conduct of an evaluation.

66 Jane Lethbridge, 'An Introduction to Evaluation', *Community Health Action*, 1989, No. 12 (Spring), pp. 5-6.
Offers a brief summary of the main issues in evaluation for CDH projects:

who evaluation is for; ways of doing it; the quantitative versus the qualitative and how to use evaluation results.

A note on the availability of the literature cited

Many of the individual project reports that are key readings for CDH workers have had limited print runs, and they are most easily available from the Resource Centre at NCHR, for the cost of photocopying and postage. The only periodical exclusively devoted to CDH work in Britain is *Community Health Action*, the newsletter of NCHR. Articles that have appeared from time to time in other academic and professional journals on CDH subjects are also kept for reference in the NCHR Resource Centre, 15 Britannia St, London WC1Y 9JP.

Section 4: Summary

We have endeavoured in this booklet to present an overview of activity in the UK on Community Participation in Health. We have by no means included everything, but we hope this gives a flavour of the vast range of levels of activity which exists.

This way of working can seem time-consuming and creates challenges for evaluation strategies. However we believe that the process involved is as valuable as the outcome. The process is developmental, and as such work may progress into areas and activities that were not originally envisaged. This means that all parties need to be flexible and open to change, basing their work on commonly agreed principles rather than rigid goals. There is no doubt that many in positions of power will find this way of working alien. However, opportunities to work in new and innovative ways provide benefits for communities, bureaucrats and professionals alike.

'Health For All' has given us a vision and provides the impetus, through initiatives like Healthy Cities, to build new working relationships, make services more open and democratic, and to recognise the wider factors that affect health.

For us, community development is one vital way of ensuring that the vision can start to be realised in people's everyday lives.

Section 5: Key Texts: a useful starting point

A Guide to Community Health Projects

Health Education Authority/National Community Health Resource, 1988.
Available from: NCHR
　　　　　　　　15 Britannia Street
　　　　　　　　London
　　　　　　　　WC1X 9JP

Community Workers' Skills Manual

Association of Community Workers, 1981.
Available from: ACW
　　　　　　　　Grindon Lodge
　　　　　　　　Beech Grove Road
　　　　　　　　Newcàstle-Upon-Tyne
　　　　　　　　NE4 2RS

Action for Health

Health Education Authority/Community Projects Foundation, 1988.
Available from: Community Projects Foundation
　　　　　　　　60 Highbury Grove
　　　　　　　　London N5 2AG